Ketogenic Dessert

Recipes

Effective Low-Carb Recipes To Balance Hormones And Effortlessly Reach Your Weight Loss Goal.

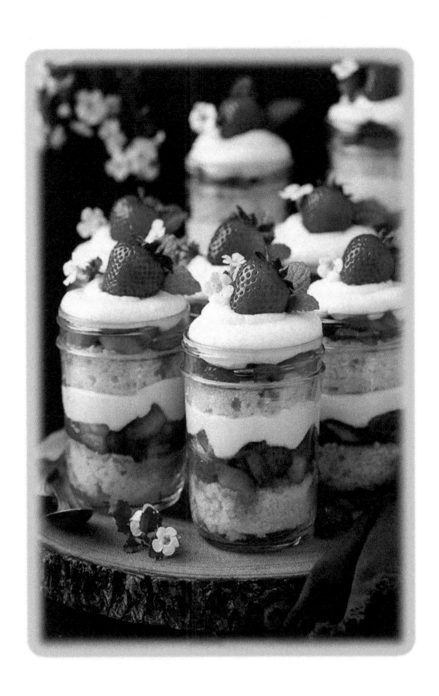

Ketogenic lifestyle...here we come!

Introduction

Do you want to make a change in your life? Do you want to become a healthier person who can enjoy a new and improved life? Then, you are definitely in the right place. You are about to discover a wonderful and very healthy diet that has changed millions of lives. We are talking about the Ketogenic diet, a lifestyle that will mesmerize you and that will make you a new person in no time.

So, let's sit back, relax and find out more about the Ketogenic diet.

A keto diet is a low carb one. This is the first and one of the most important things you should now. During such a diet, your body makes ketones in your liver and these are used as energy.

Your body will produce less insulin and glucose and a state of ketosis is induced. Ketosis is a natural process that appears when our food intake is lower than usual. The body will soon adapt to this state and therefore you will be able to lose weight in no time but you will also become healthier and your physical and mental performances will improve.

Your blood sugar levels will improve and you won't be predisposed to diabetes. Also, epilepsy and heart diseases can be prevented if you are on a Ketogenic diet.
Your cholesterol will improve and you will feel amazing in no time.

How does that sound

A Ketogenic diet is simple and easy to follow as long as you follow some simple rules. You don't need to make huge changes but there are some things you should know.
So, here goes!

Now let's start our magical culinary journey!

Ketogenic lifestyle...here we come!

Enjoy!

Tasty Chocolate Cookies

Even your kids will love these keto cookies!

Preparation time: 10 minutes **Cooking time:** 40 minutes **Servings:** 12

Ingredients:
- 1 teaspoon vanilla extract
- ½ cup ghee
- 1 egg
- 2 tablespoons coconut sugar
- ¼ cup swerve
- A pinch of salt
- 2 cups almond flour
- ½ cup unsweetened chocolate chips

Directions:
1. Heat up a pan with the ghee over medium heat, stir and cook until it browns.
2. Take this off heat and leave aside for 5 minutes.
3. In a bowl, mix egg with vanilla extract, coconut sugar and swerve and stir.
4. Add melted ghee, flour, salt and half of the chocolate chips and stir everything.
5. Transfer this to a pan, spread the rest of the chocolate chips on top, introduce in the oven at 350 degrees F and bake for 30 minutes.
6. Slice when it's cold and serve

Enjoy!

Nutrition: calories 230, fat 12, fiber 2, carbs 4, protein 5

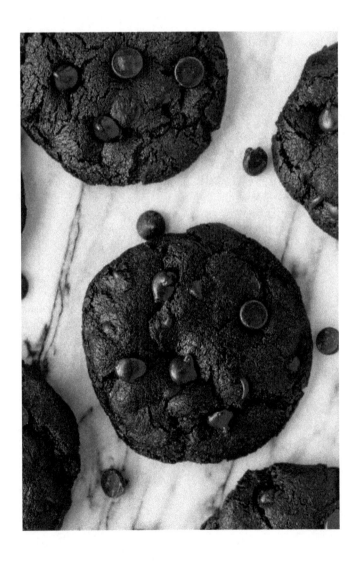

Orange Cake

You have to try this cake today!

Preparation time: 10 minutes **Cooking time:** 20 minutes **Servings:** 12

Ingredients:

- 6 eggs
- 1 orange, cut into quarters
- 1 teaspoon vanilla extract
- 1 teaspoon baking powder
- 9 ounces almond meal
- 4 tablespoons swerve
- A pinch of salt
- 2 tablespoons orange zest
- 2 ounces stevia
- 4 ounces cream cheese
- 4 ounces coconut yogurt

Directions:

1. In your food processor, pulse orange very well.
2. Add almond meal, swerve, eggs, baking powder, vanilla extract and a pinch of salt and pulse well again.
3. Transfer this into 2 spring form pans, introduce in the oven at 350 degrees F and bake for 20 minutes.
4. Meanwhile, in a bowl, mix cream cheese with orange zest, coconut yogurt and stevia and stir well.
5. Place one cake layer on a plate, add half of the cream cheese mix, add the other cake layer and top with the rest of the cream cheese mix.
6. Spread it well, slice and serve.

Enjoy!

Nutrition: calories 200, fat 13, fiber 2, carbs 5, protein 8

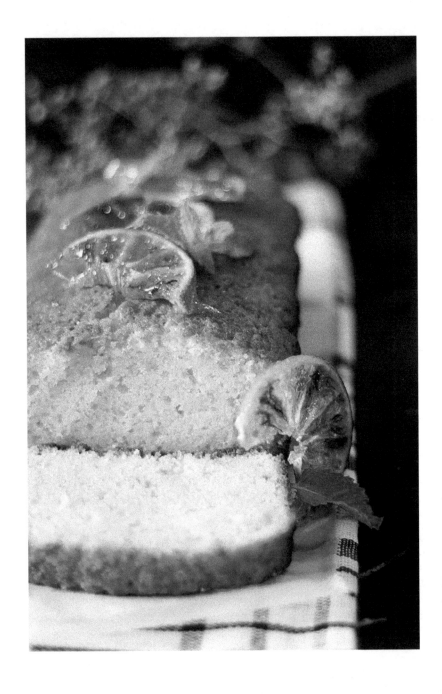

Tasty Nutella

Make your own keto nutella!

Preparation time: 10 minutes **Cooking time:** 0 minutes **Servings:** 6

Ingredients:
- 2 ounces coconut oil
- 4 tablespoons cocoa powder
- 1 teaspoon vanilla extract
- 1 cup walnuts, halved
- 4 tablespoons stevia

Directions:

1. In your food processor, mix cocoa powder with oil, vanilla, walnuts and stevia and blend very well.
2. Keep in the fridge for a couple of hours and then serve.

Enjoy!

Nutrition: calories 100, fat 10, fiber 1, carbs 3, protein 2

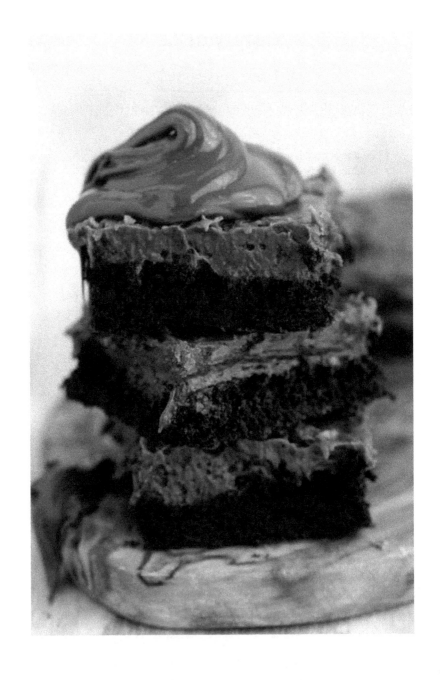

Mug Cake

This is very simple and tasty!

Preparation time: 2 minutes **Cooking time:** 3 minutes **Servings:** 1

Ingredients:
- 4 tablespoons almond meal
- 2 tablespoon ghee
- 1 teaspoon stevia
- 1 tablespoon cocoa powder, unsweetened
- 1 egg
- 1 tablespoon coconut flour
- ¼ teaspoon vanilla extract
- ½ teaspoon baking powder

Directions:
1. Put the ghee in a mug and introduce in the microwave for a couple of seconds.
2. Add cocoa powder, stevia, egg, baking powder, vanilla and coconut flour and stir well.
3. Add almond meal as well, stir again, introduce in the microwave and cook for 2 minutes.
4. Serve your mug cake with berries on top.

Enjoy!

Nutrition: calories 450, fat 34, fiber 7, carbs 10, protein 20

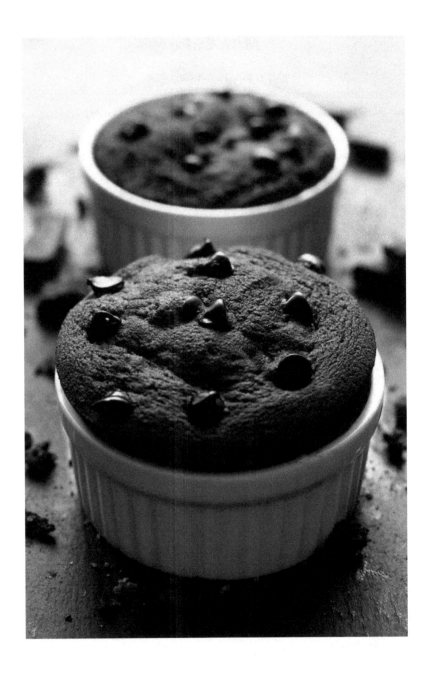

Delicious Sweet Buns

You will adore these keto buns and so will everyone else around you!

Preparation time: 10 minutes **Cooking time:** 30 minutes **Servings:** 8

Ingredients:

- ½ cup coconut flour
- 1/3 cup psyllium husks
- 2 tablespoons swerve
- 1 teaspoon baking powder
- A pinch of salt
- ½ teaspoon cinnamon
- ½ teaspoon cloves, ground
- 4 eggs
- Some chocolate chips, unsweetened
- 1 cup hot water

Directions:

1. In a bowl, mix flour with psyllium husks, swerve, baking powder, salt, cinnamon, cloves and chocolate chips and stir well.
2. Add water and egg, stir well until you obtain a dough, shape 8 buns and arrange them on a lined baking sheet.
3. Introduce in the oven at 350 degrees and bake for 30 minutes.
4. Serve these buns with some almond milk and enjoy!

Nutrition: calories 100, fat 3, fiber 3, carbs 6, protein 6

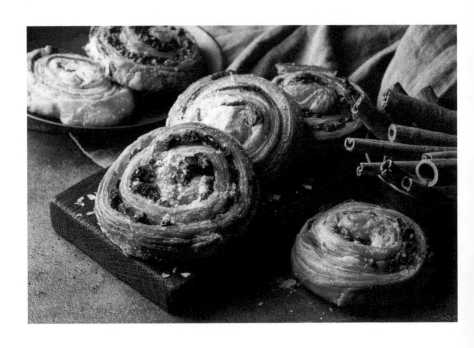

Lemon Custard

This is just irresistible!

Preparation time: 10 minutes **Cooking time:** 30 minutes **Servings:** 6

Ingredients:
- 1 and 1/3 pint almond milk
- 4 tablespoons lemon zest
- 4 eggs
- 5 tablespoons swerve
- 2 tablespoons lemon juice

Directions:

1. In a bowl, mix eggs with milk and swerve and stir very well.
2. Add lemon zest and lemon juice, whisk well, pour into ramekins and place them into a baking dish with some water on the bottom.
3. Bake in the oven at 360 degrees F for 30 minutes.
4. Leave custard to cool down before serving it.

Enjoy!

Nutrition: calories 120, fat 6, fiber 2, carbs 5, protein 7

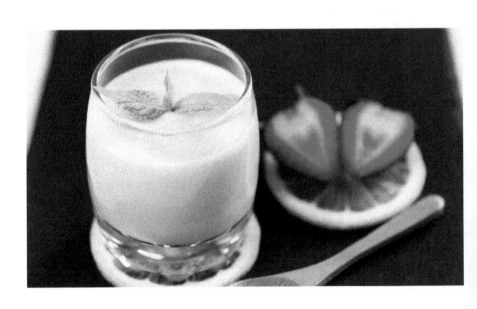

Chocolate Ganache

It will be done in 5 minutes and it's completely Ketogenic!

Preparation time: 1 minute **Cooking time:** 5 minutes **Servings:** 6

Ingredients:
- ½ cup heavy cream
- 4 ounces dark chocolate, unsweetened and chopped

Directions:
1. Put cream into a pan and heat up over medium heat.
2. Take off heat when it begins to simmer, add chocolate pieces and stir until it melts.
3. Serve this very cold as a dessert or use it as a cream for a keto cake.

Enjoy!

Nutrition: calories 78, fat 1, fiber 1, carbs 2, protein 0

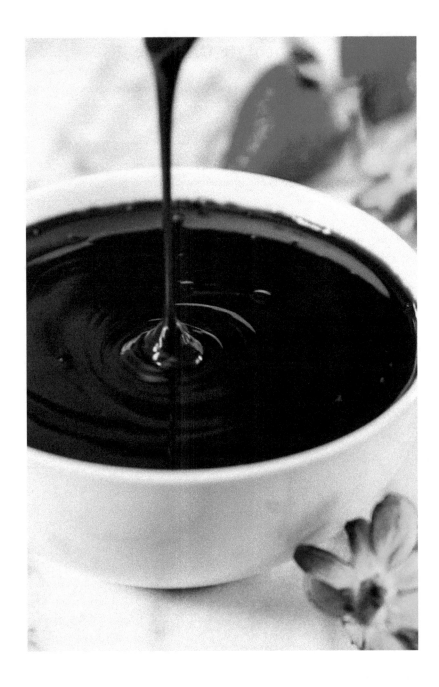

Yummy Berries Dessert

You should try a new keto dessert each day! This is our suggestion for today!

Preparation time: 10 minutes **Cooking time:** 0 minutes **Servings:** 4

Ingredients:
- 3 tablespoons cocoa powder
- 14 ounces heavy cream
- 1 cup blackberries
- 1 cup raspberries
- 2 tablespoons stevia
- Some coconut chips

Directions:
1. In a bowl, whisk cocoa powder with stevia and heavy cream.
2. Divide some of this mix into dessert bowls, add blackberries, raspberries and coconut chips, then spread another layer of cream and top with berries and chips.
3. Serve these cold.

Enjoy!

Nutrition: calories 245, fat 34, fiber 2, carbs 6, protein 2

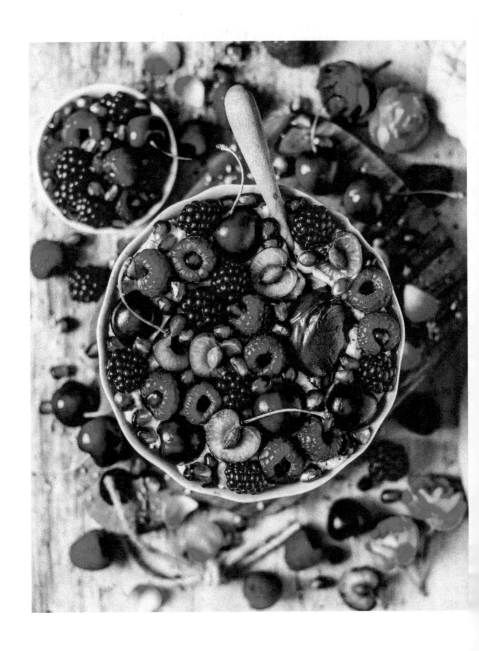

Coconut Ice Cream

It's perfect for the summer!

Preparation time: 10 minutes **Cooking time:** 0 minutes **Servings:** 4

Ingredients:
- 1 mango, sliced
- 14 ounces coconut cream, frozen

Directions:

1. In your food processor, mix mango with the cream and pulse well.

   Divide into bowls and serve right away.

Enjoy!

Nutrition: calories 150, fat 12, fiber 2, carbs 6, protein 1

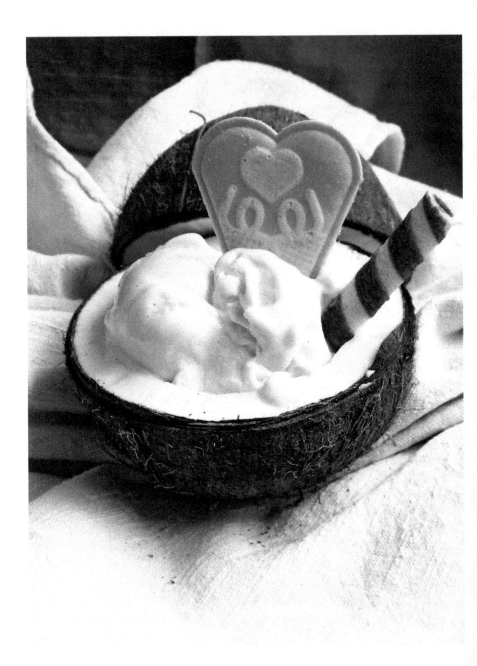

Simple Macaroons

Try these keto macaroons and enjoy them!

Preparation time: 10 minutes **Cooking time:** 10 minutes **Servings:** 20

Ingredients:

- 2 tablespoons stevia
- 4 egg whites
- 2 cup coconut, shredded
- 1 teaspoon vanilla extract

Directions:

1. In a bowl, mix egg whites with stevia and beat using your mixer.
2. Add coconut and vanilla extract and stir.
3. Roll this mix into small balls and place them on a lined baking sheet.
4. Introduce in the oven at 350 degrees F and bake for 10 minutes.
5. Serve your macaroons cold.

Enjoy!

Nutrition: calories 55, fat 6, fiber 1, carbs 2, protein 1

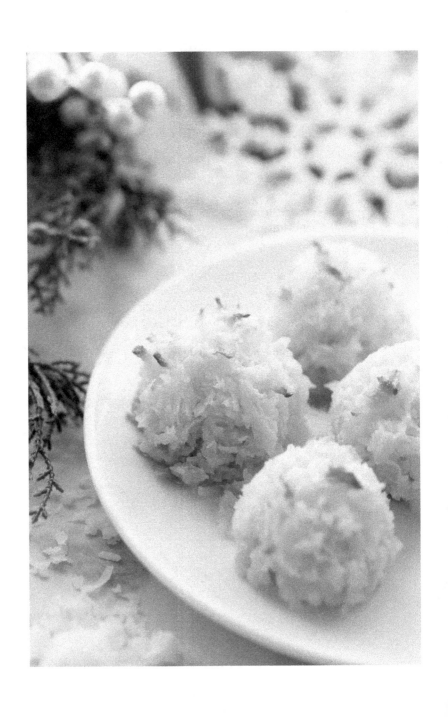

Simple Lime Cheesecake

It's the perfect cheesecake for a hot day!

Preparation time: 10 minutes **Cooking time:** 2 minutes **Servings:** 10

Ingredients:
- 2 tablespoons ghee, melted
- 2 teaspoons granulated stevia
- 4 ounces almond meal
- ¼ cup coconut, unsweetened and shredded

For the filling:
- 1 pound cream cheese
- Zest from 1 lime
- Juice from 1 lime
- 2 sachets sugar free lime jelly
- 2 cup hot water

Directions:
1. Heat up a small pan over medium heat, add ghee and stir until it melts.
2. In a bowl, mix coconut with almond meal, ghee and stevia and stir well.
3. Press this on the bottom of a round pan and keep in the fridge for now.
4. Meanwhile, put hot water in a bowl, add jelly sachets and stir until it dissolves.
5. Put cream cheese in a bowl, add jelly and stir very well.
6. Add lime juice and zest and blend using your mixer.
7. Pour this over base, spread and keep the cheesecake in the fridge until you serve it.

Enjoy!

Nutrition: calories 300, fat 23, fiber 2, carbs 5, protein 7

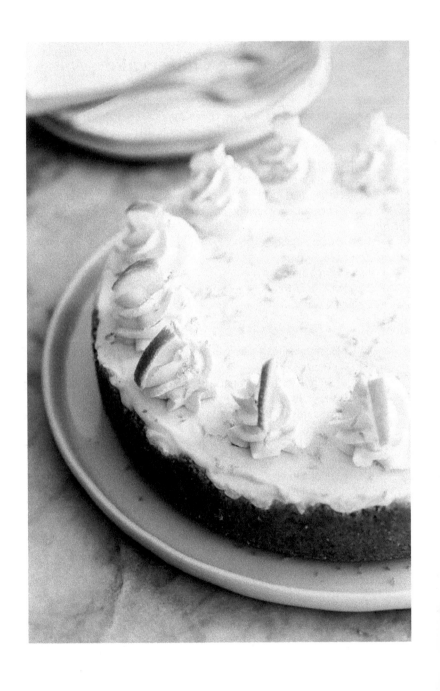

Coconut And Strawberry Delight

We won't tell you anything about this delight! Just pay attention!

Preparation time: 10 minutes **Cooking time:** 0 minutes **Servings:** 4

Ingredients:
- 1 and ¾ cups coconut cream
- 2 teaspoons granulated stevia
- 1 cup strawberries

Directions:
1. Put coconut cream in a bowl, add stevia and stir very well using an immersion blender.
2. Add strawberries, fold them gently into the mix, divide dessert into glasses and serve them cold.

Enjoy!

Nutrition: calories 245, fat 24, fiber 1, carbs 5, protein 4

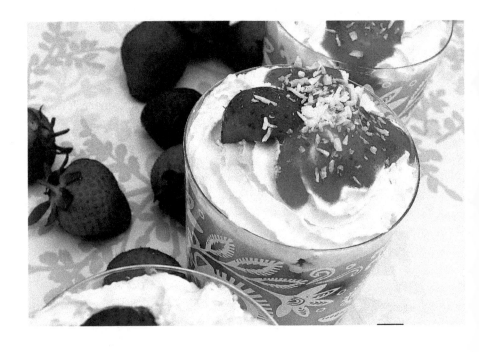

Caramel Custard

It will be done in no time!

Preparation time: 10 minutes **Cooking time:** 30 minutes **Servings:** 2

Ingredients:
- 1 and ½ teaspoons caramel extract
- 1 cup water
- 2 ounces cream cheese
- 2 eggs
- 1 and ½ tablespoons swerve

For the caramel sauce:
- 2 tablespoons swerve
- 2 tablespoons ghee
- ¼ teaspoon caramel extract

Directions:
1. In your blender, mix cream cheese with water, 1 and ½ tablespoons swerve, 1 and ½ teaspoons caramel extract and eggs and blend well.
2. Pour this into 2 greased ramekins, introduce in the oven at 350 degrees F and bake for 30 minutes.
3. Meanwhile, put the ghee in a pot and heat up over medium heat add ¼ teaspoon caramel extract and 2 tablespoons swerve, stir well and cook until everything melts.
4. Pour this over caramel custard, leave everything to cool down and serve.

Enjoy!

Nutrition: calories 254, fat 24, fiber 1, carbs 2, protein 8

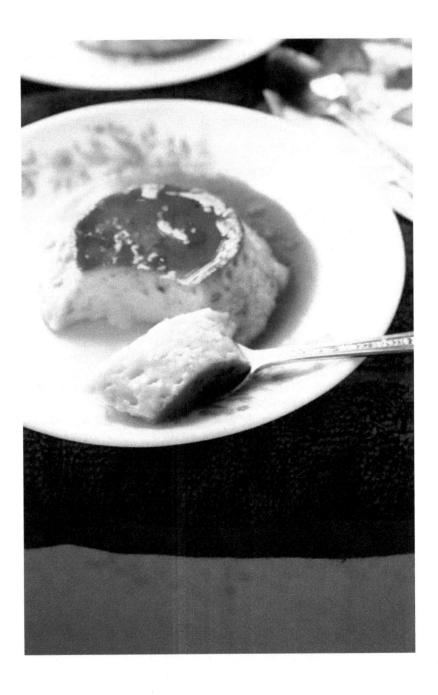

Cookie Dough Balls

These are so amazing and delicious!

Preparation time: 10 minutes **Cooking time:** 0 minutes **Servings:** 10

Ingredients:
- ½ cup almond butter
- 3 tablespoons coconut flour
- 3 tablespoons coconut milk
- 1 teaspoon cinnamon, powder
- 3 tablespoons coconut sugar
- 15 drops vanilla stevia
- A pinch of salt
- ½ teaspoon vanilla extract

For the topping:
- 1 and ½ teaspoon cinnamon powder
- 3 tablespoons granulated swerve

Directions:
1. In a bowl, mix almond butter with 1 teaspoon cinnamon, coconut flour, coconut milk, coconut sugar, vanilla extract, vanilla stevia and a pinch of salt and stir well.
2. Shape balls out of this mix.
3. In another bowl mix 1 and ½ teaspoon cinnamon powder with swerve and stir well.
4. Roll balls in cinnamon mix and keep them in the fridge until you serve.

Enjoy!

Nutrition: calories 89, fat 1, fiber 2, carbs 4, protein 2

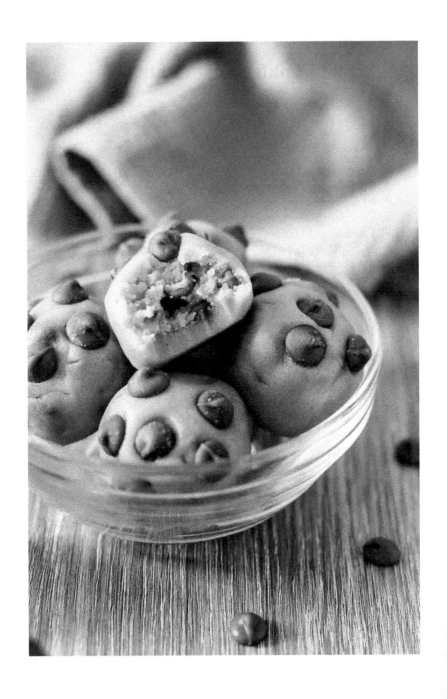

Ricotta Mousse

Serve this cold and enjoy!

Preparation time: 2 hours and 10 minutes **Cooking time:** 0 minutes **Servings:** 10

Ingredients:

- ½ cup hot coffee
- 2 cups ricotta cheese
- 2 and ½ teaspoons gelatin
- 1 teaspoon vanilla extract
- 1 teaspoon espresso powder
- 1 teaspoon vanilla stevia
- A pinch of salt
- 1 cup whipping cream

Directions:

1. In a bowl, mix coffee with gelatin, stir well and leave aside until coffee is cold.
2. In a bowl, mix espresso, stevia, salt, vanilla extract and ricotta and stir using a mixer.
3. Add coffee mix and stir everything well.
4. Add whipping cream and blend mixture again.
5. Divide into dessert bowls and serve after you've kept it in the fridge for 2 hours.

Enjoy!

Nutrition: calories 160, fat 13, fiber 0, carbs 2, protein 7

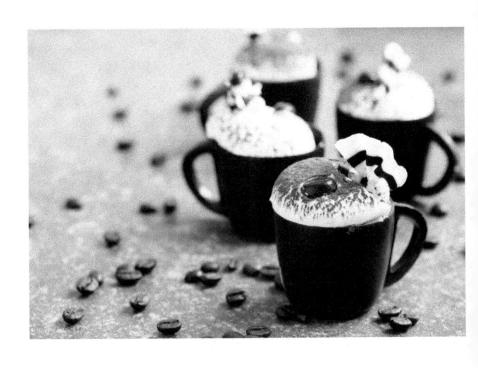

Dessert Granola

It's more than you could expect!

Preparation time: 10 minutes **Cooking time:** 35 minutes **Servings:** 4

Ingredients:
- 1 cup coconut, unsweetened and shredded
- 1 cup almonds and pecans, chopped
- 2 tablespoons stevia
- ½ cup pumpkin seeds
- ½ cup sunflower seeds
- 2 tablespoons coconut oil
- 1 teaspoon nutmeg, ground
- 1 teaspoon apple pie spice mix

Directions:
1. In a bowl, mix almonds and pecans with pumpkin seeds, sunflower seeds, coconut, nutmeg and apple pie spice mix and stir well.
2. Heat up a pan with the coconut oil over medium heat, add stevia and stir until they combine.
3. Pour this over nuts and coconut mix and stir well.
4. Spread this on a lined baking sheet, introduce in the oven at 300 degrees F and bake for 30 minutes.
5. Leave your granola to cool down, cut and serve it.

Enjoy!

Nutrition: calories 120, fat 2, fiber 2, carbs 4, protein 7

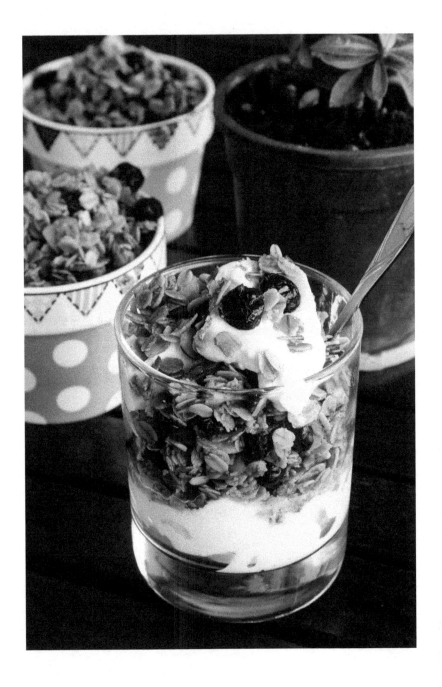

Amazing Peanut Butter And Chia Pudding

The combination is very delicious!

Preparation time: 10 minutes **Cooking time:** 0 minutes **Servings:** 4

Ingredients:
- ½ cup chia seeds
- 2 cups almond milk, unsweetened
- 1 teaspoon vanilla extract
- ¼ cup peanut butter, unsweetened
- 1 teaspoon vanilla stevia
- A pinch of salt

Directions:

1. In a bowl, mix milk with chia seeds, peanut butter, vanilla extract, stevia and pinch of salt and stir well.
2. Leave this pudding aside for 5 minutes, then stir it again, divide into dessert glasses and leave in the fridge for 10 minutes.

Enjoy!

Nutrition: calories 120, fat 1, fiber 2, carbs 4, protein 2

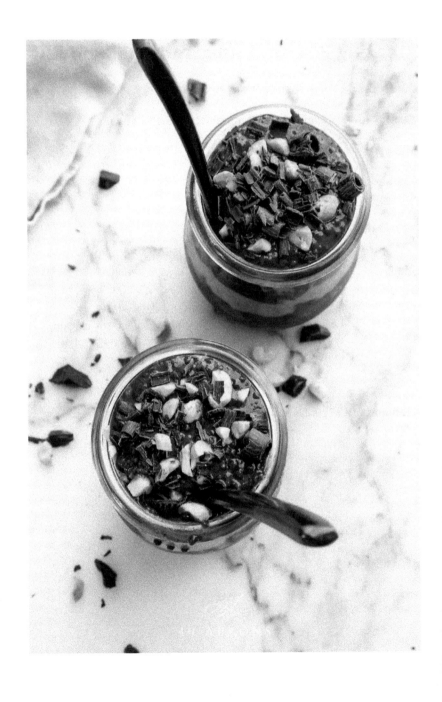

Tasty Pumpkin Custard

It's one of our favorite keto desserts! Try it today!

Preparation time: 10 minutes **Cooking time:** 5 minutes **Servings:** 6

Ingredients:

- 1 tablespoon gelatin
- ¼ cup warm water
- 14 ounces canned coconut milk
- 14 ounces canned pumpkin puree
- A pinch of salt
- 2 teaspoons vanilla extract
- 1 teaspoon cinnamon powder
- 1 teaspoon pumpkin pie spice
- 8 scoops stevia
- 3 tablespoons erythritol

Directions:

1. In a pot, mix pumpkin puree with coconut milk, a pinch of salt, vanilla extract, cinnamon powder, stevia, erythritol and pumpkin pie spice, stir well and heat up for a couple of minutes.
2. In a bowl, mix gelatin and water and stir.
3. Combine the 2 mixtures, stir well, divide custard into ramekins and leave aside to cool down.
4. Keep in the fridge until you serve it.

Enjoy!

Nutrition: calories 200, fat 2, fiber 1, carbs 3, protein 5

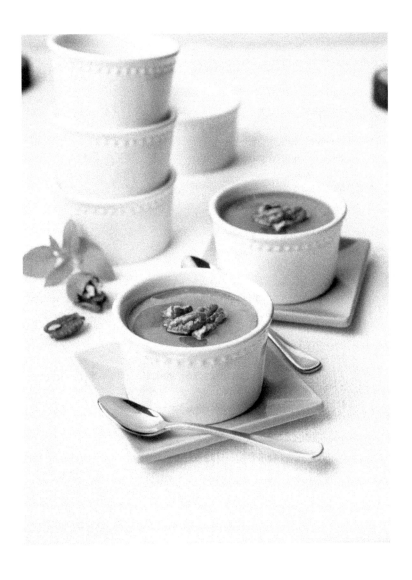

No Bake Cookies

These are stunning and so yummy!

Preparation time: 40 minutes **Cooking time:** 2 minutes **Servings:** 4

Ingredients:
- 1 cup swerve
- ¼ cup coconut milk
- ¼ cup coconut oil
- 2 tablespoons cocoa powder
- 1 and ¾ cup coconut, shredded
- ½ teaspoon vanilla extract
- A pinch of salt
- ¾ cup almond butter

Directions:

1. Heat up a pan with the oil over medium high heat, add milk, cocoa powder and swerve, stir well for about 2 minutes and take off heat.
2. Add vanilla, a pinch of salt, coconut and almond butter and stir very well.
3. Place spoonful of this mix on a lined baking sheet, keep in the fridge for 30 minutes and then serve them.

Enjoy!

Nutrition: calories 150, fat 2, fiber 1, carbs 3, protein 6

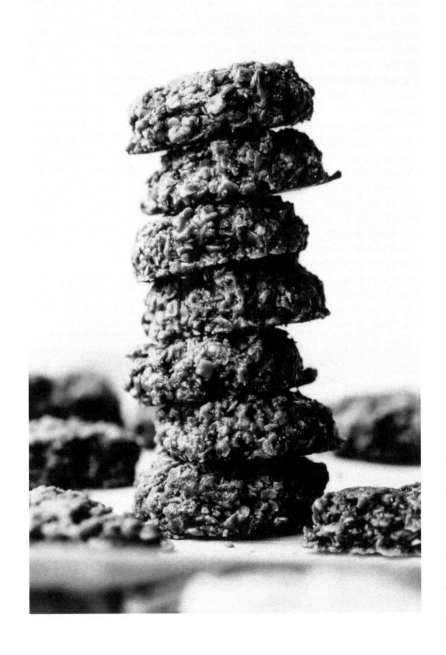

Butter Delight

It not just tasty! It also looks amazing!

Preparation time: 10 minutes **Cooking time:** 4 minutes **Servings:** 16

Ingredients:

- 4 ounces coconut butter
- 4 ounces cocoa butter
- ¼ cup swerve
- ½ cup peanut butter
- 4 ounces dark chocolate, sugar free
- ½ teaspoon vanilla extract
- 1/8 teaspoon xanthan gum

Directions:

1. Put all butter and swerve in a pan and heat up over medium heat.
2. Stir until they all combine and then mix with xanthan gum and vanilla extract.
3. Stir well again, pour into a lined baking sheet and spread well.
4. Keep this in the fridge for 10 minutes.
5. Heat up a pan with water over medium high heat and bring to a simmer.
6. Add a bowl on top of the pan and add chocolate to the bowl.
7. Stir until it melts and drizzle this over butter mix.
8. Keep in the fridge until everything is firm, cut into 16 pieces and serve.

Enjoy!

Nutrition: calories 176, fat 15, fiber 2, carbs 5, protein 3

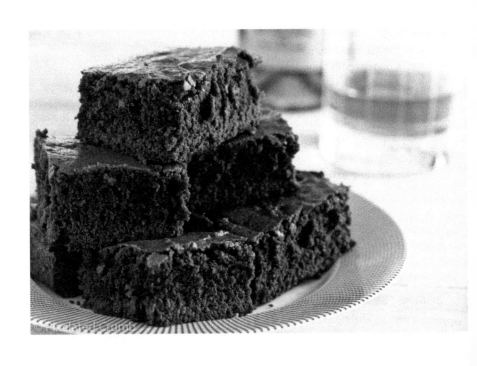

Tasty Marshmallows

Did you know you can make the keto version at home?

Preparation time: 10 minutes **Cooking time:** 3 minutes **Servings:** 6

Ingredients:

- 2 tablespoons gelatin
- 12 scoops stevia
- ½ cup cold water
- ½ cup hot water
- 2 teaspoons vanilla extract
- ¾ cup erythritol

Directions:

1. In a bowl, mix gelatin with cold water, stir and leave aside for 5 minutes.
2. Put hot water in a pan, add erythritol and stevia and stir well.
3. Combine this with the gelatin mix, add vanilla extract and stir everything well.
4. Beat this using a mixer and pour into a baking pan.
5. Leave aside in the fridge until it sets, then cut into pieces and serve.

Enjoy!

Nutrition: calories 140, fat 2, fiber 1, carbs 2, protein 4

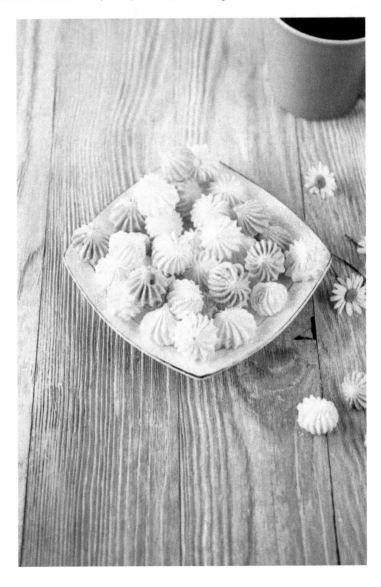

Delicious Tiramisu Pudding

Try a keto tiramisu pudding today!

Preparation time: 2 hours and 10 minutes **Cooking time:** 0 minutes **Servings:** 1

Ingredients:

- 8 ounces cream cheese
- 16 ounces cottage cheese
- 2 tablespoons cocoa powder
- 1 teaspoon instant coffee
- 4 tablespoons almond milk
- 1 and ½ cup splenda

Directions:

1. In your food processor, mix cottage cheese with cream cheese, cocoa powder and coffee and blend very well.
2. Add splenda and almond milk, blend again and divide into dessert cups.
3. Keep in the fridge until you serve.

Enjoy!

Nutrition: calories 200, fat 2, fiber 2, carbs 5, protein 5

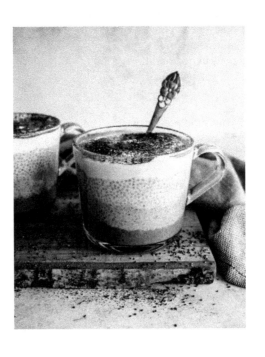

Summer Dessert Smoothie

It's easy and super refreshing! You can try it today!

Preparation time: 5 minutes **Cooking time:** 0 minutes **Servings:** 2

Ingredients:

- ½ cup coconut milk
- 1 and ½ cup avocado, pitted and peeled
- 2 tablespoons green tea powder
- 2 teaspoons lime zest
- 1 tablespoon coconut sugar
- 1 mango thinly sliced for serving

Directions:

1. In your smoothie maker, combine milk with avocado, green tea powder and lime zest and pulse well.
2. Add sugar, blend well, divide into 2 glasses and serve with mango slices on top.

Enjoy!

Nutrition: calories 87, fat 5, fiber 3, carbs 6, protein 8

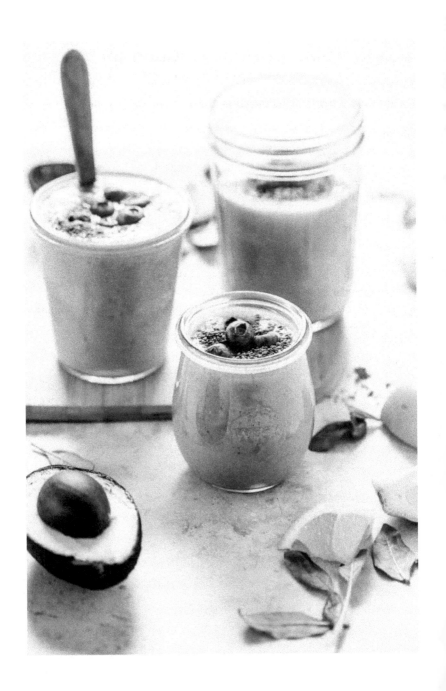

Lemon Sorbet

You only need 3 ingredients t\om make this cool and keto dessert!

Preparation time: 5 minutes **Cooking time:** 0 minutes **Servings:** 4

Ingredients:
- 4 cups ice
- Stevia to the taste
- 1 lemon, peeled and roughly chopped

Directions :

1. In your blender, mix lemon piece with stevia and ice and blend until everything is combined.
2. Divide into glasses and serve very cold.

Enjoy!

Nutrition: calories 67, fat 0, fiber 0, carbs 1, protein 1

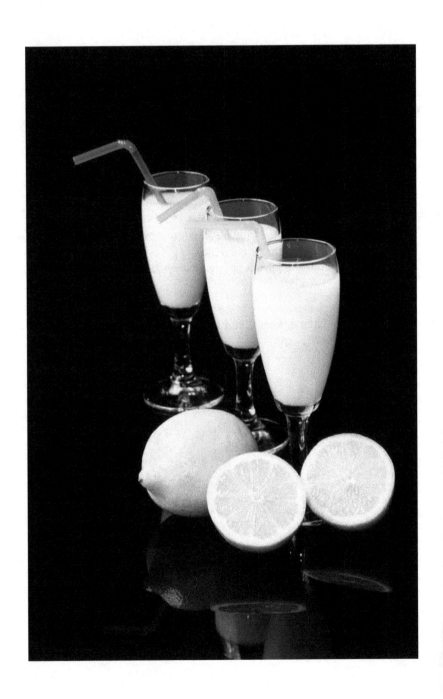

Simple Raspberry Popsicles

It can't get any easier than this! You basically only need one ingredients: raspberries!

Preparation time: 2 hours **Cooking time:** 10 minutes **Servings:** 4

Ingredients:
- 1 and ½ cups raspberries
- 2 cups water

Directions:
1. Put raspberries and water in a pan, bring to a boil and simmer for 10 minutes at a medium temperature.
2. Pour mix in an ice cube tray, stick popsicles sticks in each and chill in the freezer for 2 hours.

Enjoy!

Nutrition: calories 60, fat 0, fiber 0, carbs 0, protein 2

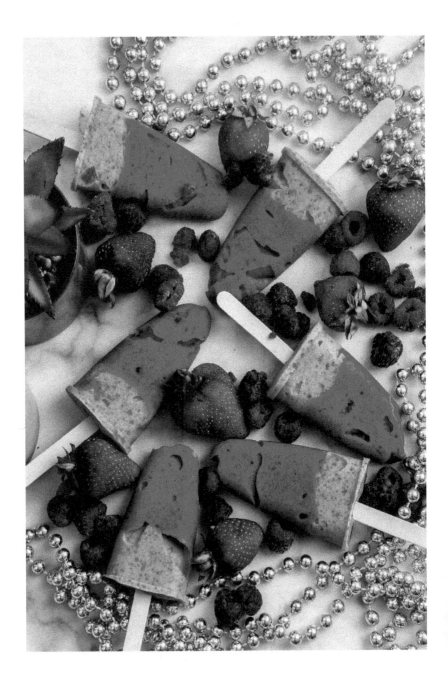

Cherry And Chia Jam

Your family will love this great keto dessert!

Preparation time: 15 minutes **Cooking time:** 12 minutes **Servings:** 22

Ingredients:

- 3 tablespoons chia seeds
- 2 and ½ cups cherries, pitted
- ½ teaspoon vanilla powder
- Peel from ½ lemon, grated
- ¼ cup erythritol
- 10 drops stevia
- 1 cup water

Directions:

1. Put cherries and the water in a pot, add stevia, erythritol, vanilla powder, chia seeds and lemon peel, stir, bring to a simmer and cook for 12 minutes.
2. Take off heat and leave your jam aside for 15 minutes at least.
3. Serve cold.

Enjoy!

Nutrition: calories 60, fat 1, fiber 1, carbs 2, protein 0.5

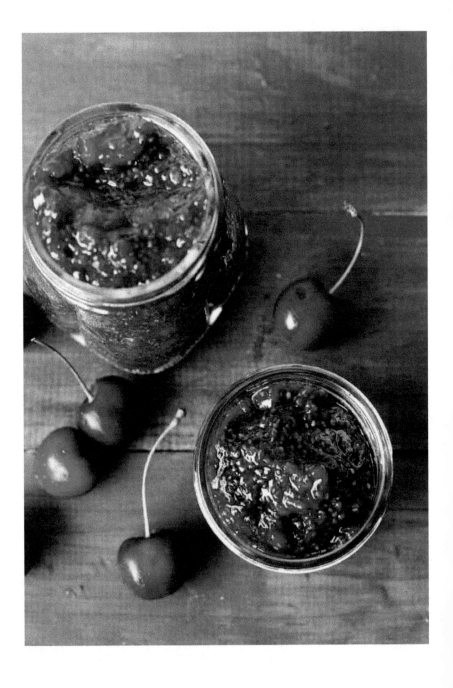

Amazing Jello Dessert

It's more than you can imagine!

Preparation time: 2 hours 10 minutes **Cooking time:** 5 minutes **Servings:** 12

Ingredients:
- 2 ounces packets sugar free jello
- 1 cup cold water
- 1 cup hot water
- 3 tablespoons erythritol
- 2 tablespoons gelatin powder
- 1 teaspoon vanilla extract
- 1 cup heavy cream
- 1 cup boiling water

Directions:
1. Put jello packets in a bowl, add 1 cup hot water, stir until it dissolves and then mix with 1 cup cold water.
2. Pour this into a lined square dish and keep in the fridge for 1 hour.
3. Cut into cubes and leave aside for now.
4. Meanwhile, in a bowl, mix erythritol with vanilla extract, 1 cup boiling water, gelatin and heavy cream and stir very well.
5. Pour half of this mix into a silicon round mold, spread jello cubes, then top with the rest of the gelatin.
6. Keep in the fridge for 1 more hour and then serve.

Enjoy!

Nutrition: calories 70, fat 1, fiber 0, carbs 1, protein 2

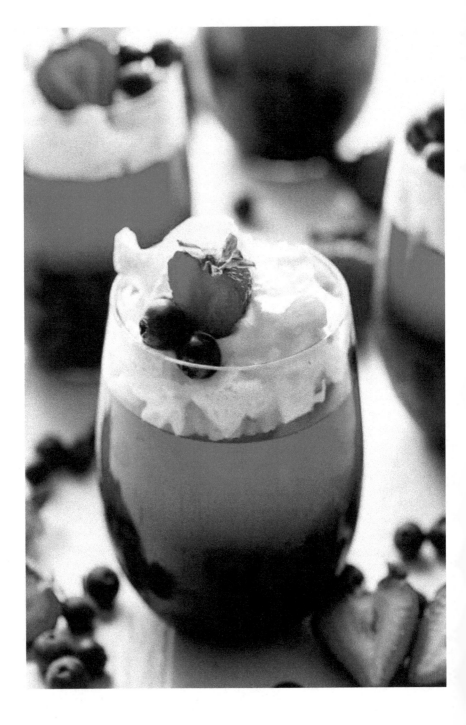

Strawberry Pie

It's so delicious!

Preparation time: 2 hours and 10 minutes **Cooking time:** 5 minutes **Servings:** 12

Ingredients: *For the crust:*
- 1 cup coconut, shredded
- 1 cup sunflower seeds
- ¼ cup butter
- A pinch of salt

For the filling:
- 1 teaspoon gelatin
- 8 ounces cream cheese
- 4 ounces strawberries
- 2 tablespoons water
- ½ tablespoon lemon juice
- ¼ teaspoon stevia
- ½ cup heavy cream
- 8 ounces strawberries, chopped for serving
- 16 ounces heavy cream for serving

Directions:
1. In your food processor, mix sunflower seeds with coconut, a pinch of salt and butter and stir well.
2. Put this into a greased spring form pan and press well on the bottom.
3. Heat up a pan with the water over medium heat, add gelatin, stir until it dissolves, take off heat and leave aside to cool down.
4. Add this to your food processor, mix with 4 ounces strawberries, cream cheese, lemon juice and stevia and blend well.
5. Add ½ cup heavy cream, stir well and spread this over crust.
6. Top with 8 ounces strawberries and 16 ounces heavy cream and keep in the fridge for 2 hours before slicing and serving.

Enjoy!

Nutrition: calories 234, fat 23, fiber 2, carbs 6, protein 7

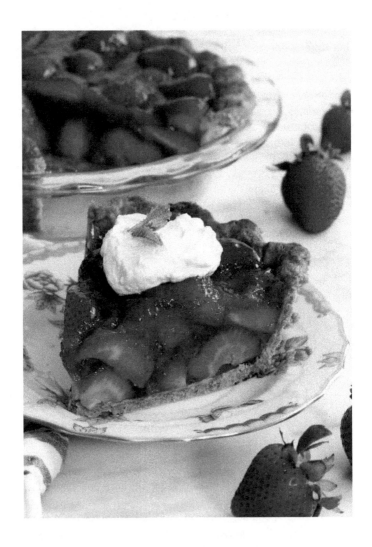

Lemon Mousse

This is so refreshing and delicious!

Preparation time: 10 minutes **Cooking time:** 0 minutes **Servings:** 5

Ingredients:

- 1 cup heavy cream
- A pinch of salt
- 1 teaspoon lemon stevia
- ¼ cup lemon juice
- 8 ounces mascarpone cheese

Directions:

1. In a bowl, mix heavy cream with mascarpone and lemon juice and stir using your mixer.
2. Add a pinch of salt and stevia and blend everything.
3. Divide into dessert glasses and keep in the fridge until you serve.

Enjoy!

Nutrition: calories 265, fat 27, fiber 0, carbs 2, protein 4

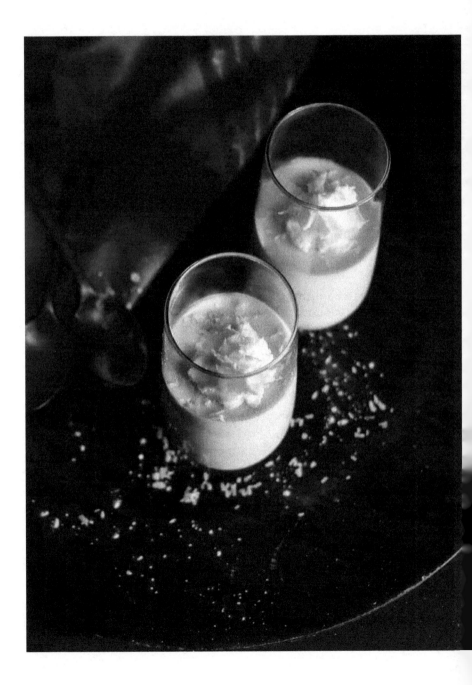

Vanilla Ice Cream

Try this keto ice cream on a summer day!

Preparation time: 3 hours and 10 minutes **Cooking time:** 0 minutes **Servings:** 6

Ingredients:

- 4 eggs, yolks and whites separated
- ¼ teaspoon cream of tartar
- ½ cup swerve
- 1 tablespoon vanilla extract
- 1 and ¼ cup heavy whipping cream

Directions:

1. In a bowl, mix egg whites with cream of tartar and swerve and stir using your mixer.
2. In another bowl, whisk cream with vanilla extract and blend very well.
3. Combine the 2 mixtures and stir gently.
4. In another bowl, whisk egg yolks very well and then add the two egg whites mix.
5. Stir gently, pour this into a container and keep in the freezer for 3 hours before serving your ice cream.

Enjoy!

Nutrition: calories 243, fat 22, fiber 0, carbs 2, protein 4

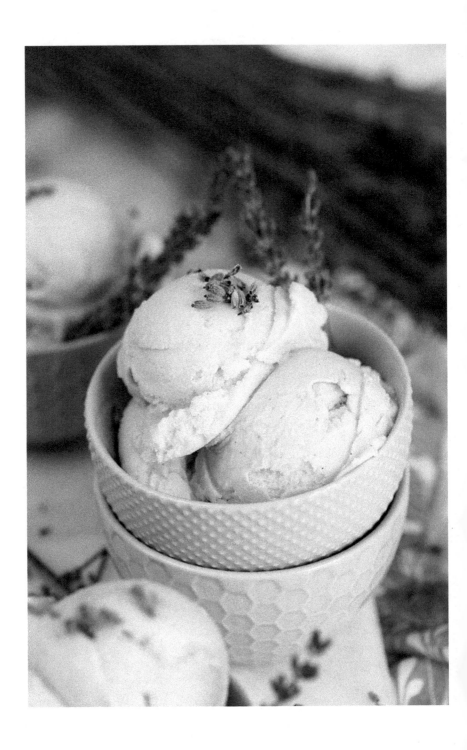

Cheesecake Squares

They look so good!

Preparation time: 10 minutes **Cooking time:** 20 minutes **Servings:** 9

Ingredients:
- 5 ounces coconut oil, melted
- ½ teaspoon baking powder
- 4 tablespoons swerve
- 1 teaspoon vanilla
- 4 ounces cream cheese
- 6 eggs
- ½ cup blueberries

Directions:

1. In a bowl, mix coconut oil with eggs, cream cheese, vanilla, swerve and baking powder and blend using an immersion blender.
2. Fold blueberries, pour everything into a square baking dish, introduce in the oven at 320 degrees F and bake for 20 minutes.
3. Leave you cake to cool down, slice into squares and serve.

Enjoy!

Nutrition: calories 220, fat 2, fiber 0.5, carbs 2, protein 4

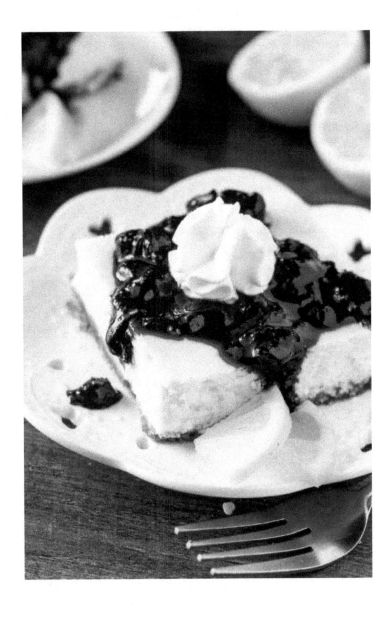

Conclusion

This is really a life changing cookbook. It shows you everything you need to know about the Ketogenic diet and it helps you get started.

You now know some of the best and most popular Ketogenic recipes in the world.

We have something for everyone's taste!

So, don't hesitate too much and start your new life as a follower of the Ketogenic diet!

Get your hands on this special recipes collection and start cooking in this new, exciting and healthy way!

Have a lot of fun and enjoy your Ketogenic diet!

Lightning Source UK Ltd.
Milton Keynes UK
UKHW020704130521
383649UK00005B/125

9 781802 870373